Walking Like Yourself Again After Knee Replacement ™

Why Walking Feels Awkward and How People Rebuild Smooth, Confident Walking for Everyday Life

Michelle Losurdo, PT, DPT, OCS

Creator and Host of the Total Knee Success Podcast™

Pale Blue Press LLC

Published by: Pale Blue Press LLC
ISBN: 978-0-9963877-4-3
Paperback Edition
Printed in the United States of America.

IMPORTANT DISCLAIMER

This book is intended for educational and informational purposes only.

It is not medical advice, diagnosis, or treatment and should not be relied upon as a substitute for individualized medical care from qualified healthcare professionals. The information presented reflects general educational principles related to knee replacement rehabilitation after surgery. Individual experiences, symptoms, medical histories, and rehabilitation responses can vary significantly.

Readers should consult their physicians, physical therapists, or other qualified healthcare providers regarding their individual situation and before making decisions related to medical care, activity, exercise, medications, or treatment.

The author and publisher disclaim responsibility for any adverse effects or consequences resulting directly or indirectly from the use of the information contained in this book.

If you experience worsening symptoms, increasing redness, warmth, drainage, fever, chest pain, sudden shortness of breath, or other urgent medical concerns, seek immediate medical attention.

Table Of Contents

INTRODUCTION

Most people expect pain, swelling, and stiffness after knee replacement. What often catches people off guard is how different walking can feel once they begin moving around more.

Most people expect to limp early after surgery. What becomes more frustrating is when movement still feels awkward, inconsistent, tiring, or unnatural longer than expected.

Movement that once felt automatic may suddenly require more thought and effort.

Some people notice they start slowing their pace, paying closer attention to uneven ground, scanning for benches during longer outings, or wondering whether they can comfortably keep up with the people around them.

A simple trip through a grocery store or parking lot can start feeling very different than it used to.

Take someone like Carol.

Carol is 68 years old. Before surgery, she stayed active, walked regularly with friends, and helped care for her grandchildren. After surgery, she expected things to improve steadily from week to week, but instead she noticed her movement quality seemed to change from one day to the next.

Some days she walked fairly comfortably around the house, while other days she developed a noticeable limp after only ten minutes on her feet. At times she felt stiff and uneven, and at other times she felt uncertain or unstable, especially on stairs, uneven ground, or when trying to keep pace with other people.

One thing that bothered her more than she expected was realizing she could not keep up with other people comfortably anymore. Walking beside friends or family suddenly felt different, and she noticed herself asking people to slow down, falling slightly behind during outings, or avoiding longer walks altogether.

What frustrated her most was not simply the discomfort itself, but the uncertainty around what she was experiencing.

She found herself wondering why she still limped so much some days, whether she should still be using the cane even though she disliked relying on it, and why her movement seemed to fall apart once she became tired.

Carol is not a real person. She is an example created to represent common experiences many people report after knee replacement.

Some parts of Carol's experience may feel familiar to you. Other people notice different challenges after surgery. Some struggle more with stiffness and swelling. Others become frustrated by limping, fatigue, balance concerns, difficulty keeping up with other people, or feeling less confident walking in public.

Walking rarely improves in a perfectly straight line. A good walking day may suddenly be followed by stiffness, fatigue, swelling, or limping the next day.

Understanding these patterns can help people stop overanalyzing every difficult walking day.

Movement after surgery usually improves when rhythm, endurance, strength, and confidence begin working together again instead of feeling disconnected from each other. Over time, people often start recognizing patterns instead of feeling like every difficult day means something has gone wrong.

Throughout this guide, we will look at:

- Why walking can still feel awkward weeks or months after surgery
- How swelling, fatigue, and limping change throughout the day
- What smoother walking mechanics actually require
- Confidence, cane use, stairs, and outdoor walking
- Rebuilding endurance for everyday life again

The goal is to help you better understand these patterns so walking gradually begins feeling smoother, steadier, and more automatic.

Why Walking Feels So Strange After Knee Replacement

It is common to assume movement should feel natural once your arthritic joint has been replaced. Instead, it often feels stiff, robotic, uneven, unstable, or exhausting during the early stages after surgery.

Several different factors are influencing movement at the same time. Swelling changes mechanics, pain changes weight distribution, weakness affects stability and control, and fatigue often makes movement less fluid.

Walking often becomes more cautious as a result.

Carol noticed this almost immediately. She shortened her stride, leaned away from the pain, and stopped swinging her arms normally. Instead of walking naturally, she began carefully managing every step, and the more attention she paid to walking, the less fluid it felt.

Almost everyone notices some version of this during the first stages of walking again.

A protective walking pattern often develops over time. The goal of this pattern is not efficiency. People often begin changing the way they move to reduce discomfort, stiffness, instability, and uncertainty while everything still feels unfamiliar.

For that reason, limping is often influenced by far more than simple weakness alone.

Several different factors can influence walking after knee replacement, including:

- Stiffness
- Swelling
- Fatigue
- Protective movement patterns
- Hesitation during weight bearing
- Balance changes
- Discomfort during weight bearing

Understanding this can help people realize that awkward or uneven walking does not automatically mean something is wrong. In many cases, it reflects your body adapting to a major physical event while gradually rebuilding tolerance and confidence.

The Protective Limp

One of the most frustrating parts of walking after knee replacement is the limp that seems to appear even when people are trying very hard to walk correctly.

Many individuals immediately assume limping means they are damaging the implant, failing rehabilitation, or walking incorrectly. In reality, limping is often your body's attempt to protect itself while strength, confidence, swelling, and movement quality are still improving.

Carol found that her limp became much more noticeable later in the day. If she stayed on her feet too long, rushed through errands, or spent too much time standing in one place, her gait gradually became more uneven. The first several steps after sitting also often felt stiff and awkward.

Over time, certain patterns became easier to recognize. Fatigue often made her movements less steady. Other days, swelling had gradually built up, or she found herself moving more cautiously because she still did not fully trust her leg.

Movement often feels smoother earlier in the day, after short movement breaks, or during shorter outings before fatigue and swelling build up.

Changes like these often become more noticeable:

- Later in the day after activity accumulates
- After long-standing periods or errands
- When rushing to keep pace with other people
- In crowded or unfamiliar environments
- During periods of increased swelling or fatigue

Recognizing these patterns can help reduce the fear some people feel when limping appears. In many cases, the body is responding to accumulated stress, fatigue, swelling, or reduced confidence rather than structural damage.

As Carol became more aware of these patterns, she stopped viewing every difficult walking day as a sign that something was wrong. Instead, she began adjusting her activity more thoughtfully and paying closer attention to how fatigue, swelling, and longer days on her feet affected her movement. That shift made difficult walking days feel easier to understand and less discouraging.

Why Persistent Limping Should Not Be Ignored

Temporary limping and walking changes are extremely common after knee replacement, especially while swelling, weakness, stiffness, fatigue, and confidence are still improving.

At the same time, persistent limping is usually something people want to gradually improve rather than simply accept long term.

Walking with significant compensations over long periods can sometimes contribute to:

- Increased fatigue
- Hip pain
- Back discomfort
- Strain on the opposite leg
- Reduced walking efficiency
- Balance problems
- Reduced endurance during daily activities

This does not mean every temporary limp is harmful or dangerous. In many cases, gait changes improve gradually as strength, endurance, swelling control, balance, and confidence continue improving over time.

The goal is usually not perfect walking mechanics. More often, the goal is smoother, more efficient movement that allows people to participate more comfortably and confidently in everyday life.

This does not mean persistent walking problems should automatically be ignored. Ongoing stiffness, major motion loss, arthrofibrosis (excessive scar tissue causing abnormal stiffness), persistent weakness, or worsening gait problems should still be discussed with your surgeon.

Why Swelling Changes Walking

Swelling is one of the biggest reasons walking changes after surgery, and it affects gait far more dramatically than most people expect.

Swelling does not just change appearance. Walking often feels heavier, stiffer, more tiring, and less natural when swelling builds up. Steps may suddenly feel awkward or uneven even on days when pain is relatively manageable.

Carol noticed that when her knee was more swollen, walking felt slower and more effortful. Movement felt tighter, less responsive, and harder to fully straighten during longer walks. She also noticed that swelling changed her confidence. When movement felt heavy or restricted, she automatically became more cautious.

Swelling commonly affects:

- Knee bending and straightening during walking
- Muscle activation and balance
- Endurance during longer outings
- Confidence during weight bearing

Pain did not always increase significantly on those days. Movement often felt heavier, stiffer, and more tiring. In many cases, swelling affects movement quality before pain changes significantly.

Movement quality frequently improves when swelling becomes more controlled through pacing, position changes, shorter activity bursts, and more consistent day-to-day activity levels.

As swelling becomes easier to manage, walking often starts feeling smoother, steadier, and less tiring.

Some swelling after knee replacement is extremely common, especially during the earlier stages after surgery or after heavier activity. Persistent swelling, worsening swelling, or swelling that continues limiting motion and walking over time should still be discussed with your surgeon.

Why Fatigue Changes Walking

Fatigue changes movement quality far more than most people expect.

Movement may feel fairly normal at first, then gradually become more awkward as muscles tire. The beginning of a grocery store trip may feel manageable, while the later part of the trip suddenly feels much harder.

Carol noticed that fatigue affected her daily life more than she expected. She could walk reasonably comfortably during the first part of an outing, then suddenly realize she was becoming much more tired and struggling to continue comfortably. By that point she was often looking for somewhere to sit, cutting errands short, or feeling too drained to do much afterward.

As muscles tire, walking often becomes stiffer, slower, and less coordinated. Arm swing decreases, balance becomes less automatic, and compensation patterns gradually increase.

Common fatigue patterns include:

- Limping later in the day
- Shorter stride length during longer walks
- More leaning or shifting during walking
- Increased stiffness after standing too long
- Reduced confidence once tired

This is one reason shorter, repeatable walking sessions often work better than exhausting yourself during occasional "good days." Walking quality usually improves more steadily when activity builds gradually instead of swinging between overactivity and exhaustion.

Rebuilding A Smoother Walking Pattern

Rebuilding smoother walking becomes much easier once people understand what normally happens during each step.

People often try to "walk correctly" without fully understanding what normally happens during walking. Once people understand the sequence, walking often starts to feel less mysterious and less frustrating.

Physical therapists often study walking using something called gait analysis. Gait analysis simply means looking closely at how a person walks so the therapist can better understand where movement changes are happening.

One commonly used framework, associated with Rancho Los Amigos National Rehabilitation Center, breaks the walking cycle into smaller phases such as initial contact, loading response, mid-stance, terminal stance, pre-swing, initial swing, mid-swing, and terminal swing.

The terminology sounds technical, but the overall walking pattern is easier to recognize once it is broken down step by step.

Walking is a repeating sequence where you:

- Accept weight
- Balance on one leg while the other leg swings forward
- Push off and move into the next step

- Repeat the same sequence with the opposite leg

The body performs this sequence thousands of times every day.

After knee replacement, the sequence often becomes disrupted because of swelling, weakness, stiffness, fatigue, discomfort, reduced confidence, and changes in balance.

Understanding these phases can help people recognize why walking feels awkward and what is supposed to happen during each step.

The Basic Rhythm of Walking

Walking follows a repeating rhythm where the body shifts smoothly from one leg to the other during each step.

Human gait follows a repeating movement pattern where one leg supports the body while the other leg moves forward to prepare for the next step. When one foot lands, several things happen together:

- The body accepts weight
- The knee bends a little like a shock absorber
- The hip helps hold the body upright
- The ankle helps the body roll forward

The body then moves over that leg before the heel lifts and the toes push off the ground. After that, the other leg swings through to take the next step. That smooth rolling pattern is what creates natural walking, and when people limp after knee replacement, part of that sequence often becomes disrupted.

How the Hip, Knee, and Ankle Work Together During Walking

Normal walking requires coordination between the hip, knee, ankle, pelvis, trunk, and nervous system. Each joint has a specific job during walking, and those jobs need to happen at the right time for movement to feel smooth.

The hip helps stabilize the body and move the leg forward. The knee absorbs force and helps the body move smoothly over the leg. The ankle controls how the foot contacts the ground and helps create push-off.

If one part is stiff, weak, swollen, painful, or poorly coordinated, the entire walking pattern can change. That is one reason a problem that feels like "just a limp" may actually involve the knee, hip, ankle, balance system, confidence, fatigue, and swelling all at the same time.

The sections below simplify certain gait and movement concepts intentionally so they are easier to understand outside of a clinical setting. Normal walking is highly complex, and clinicians often analyze gait in much greater detail during formal rehabilitation and movement assessment.

Walking is commonly divided into two main phases: stance phase and swing phase. Stance phase is when the foot is on the ground supporting the body, and swing phase is when the foot is in the air moving forward to prepare for the next step. The Rancho Los Amigos system breaks those larger phases into smaller parts so clinicians can better understand where movement changes are happening.

WHAT NORMAL WALKING ACTUALLY REQUIRES

Walking on flat ground does not require extreme knee bending, but it does require the knee to move well enough at the right times. For a reasonably normal gait pattern on level surfaces, the knee generally needs to reach close to full extension, around 0°, and needs roughly 60° of flexion during the walking cycle.

Stairs, curbs, and uneven surfaces usually require more motion than level walking. Walking up and down stairs using a step-over-step pattern often requires roughly 90-120° of knee flexion depending on step height, speed, strength, balance, and individual walking mechanics. This is why some people can walk fairly well on flat ground but still feel stiff, weak, or hesitant on stairs and curbs.

Stance Phase

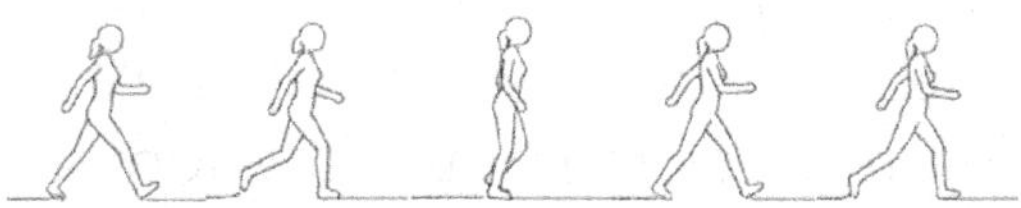

Stance phase is the part of walking when the foot is on the ground and the leg is supporting body weight. This phase includes the moment the foot first touches the ground, the transfer of weight onto the leg, the body moving over the foot, and the push-off into the next step.

After knee replacement, stance phase often feels different because the surgical leg may not feel fully trustworthy yet. Swelling, stiffness, quadriceps weakness, pain, balance changes, and hesitation during weight bearing can all make this part of walking feel cautious or uneven.

Initial Contact

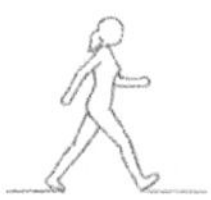

Initial contact occurs when the heel first touches the ground. During comfortable walking, the heel typically contacts first before the rest of the foot rolls down smoothly to the floor. The drawing illustrates this phase of walking, with the right leg closest to you serving as the reference leg.

At this stage of walking:

- The hip is slightly flexed
- The knee is close to straight
- The ankle is in a neutral position

The quadriceps help prepare the knee to accept weight while the hip muscles stabilize the pelvis. At the same time, the ankle prepares to control the foot as the body moves forward.

Avoiding full knee straightening during this phase is extremely common after surgery, especially when stiffness, swelling, or discomfort are still present. When the knee does not fully straighten, the ankle feels stiff, or steps become very short and cautious, people often begin landing more flat-footed instead.

That often creates:

- A bent-knee walking pattern
- Shorter stride length
- Reduced confidence during weight acceptance
- Increased limping
- A feeling of walking cautiously instead of smoothly

This is one reason some people feel slower walking beside others or notice they fatigue more quickly during longer outings.

Loading Response

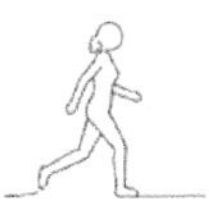

Loading response is the short period immediately after the foot touches the ground and the body begins transferring weight onto the leg. This is one of the first moments when people begin fully loading the surgical side during each step. The drawing illustrates this phase of walking, with the right leg closest to you serving as the reference leg.

During this phase:

- The hip remains slightly flexed
- The knee bends slightly, usually around 15 degrees
- The foot moves from heel contact toward a flatter position on the ground

This controlled knee bend helps absorb force more smoothly as weight transfers onto the leg. The quadriceps work hard here to control the knee while the hip muscles help stabilize the body.

This phase is important because many people after knee replacement become hesitant loading their surgical leg. If the quadriceps are weak or inhibited by swelling, the body may automatically try to reduce time spent on that side.

Common changes include:

- Shifting weight away from the surgical leg
- Leaning the trunk sideways
- Shortening stance time
- Walking cautiously

This is one reason strengthening and swelling control can make a noticeable difference in gait quality.

Mid-Stance

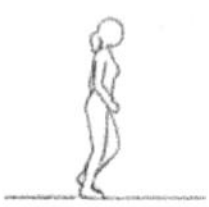

During mid-stance, the body moves directly over the leg while balance shifts onto a single limb. This is the part of walking where many people become most aware of whether they trust the surgical leg. The drawing illustrates this phase of walking, with the right leg closest to you serving as the reference leg.

At this stage of walking:

- The hip is close to a neutral standing position
- The knee should be close to fully straight

- The foot stays flat on the ground while the body moves over it

The quadriceps continue stabilizing the knee while the hip muscles help keep the pelvis level and support balance over one leg. This phase requires confidence, control, and enough strength to comfortably support the body on one side.

Many people limp most noticeably during mid-stance because they do not fully trust their leg yet. If the knee does not fully straighten during mid-stance, people often develop a bent-knee walking pattern called a flexed gait, which can increase fatigue because the muscles must work harder during every step.

Common compensations include:

- Leaning away from the surgical side
- Spending less time on the surgical leg
- Walking with incomplete knee extension
- Shortening the stride on the opposite side

People often notice these changes in real-world situations such as walking through stores, crossing parking lots, walking on uneven ground, or trying to keep pace with family members. Mid-stance is one of the clearest phases where walking confidence becomes visible.

Terminal Stance

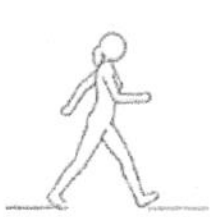

During terminal stance, the body continues moving forward over the foot while the heel begins lifting off the ground. This is where walking starts preparing for push-off into the next step. The drawing illustrates this phase of walking, with the right leg closest to you serving as the reference leg.

At this stage of walking:

- The hip extends behind the body
- The knee is generally near extension as the body moves forward, then begins preparing to bend as the leg transitions toward the next step
- The heel lifts while the toes remain on the ground

The calf muscles become very important here because they help move the body forward efficiently. When this phase is shortened, walking often becomes slower, flatter, and more effortful.

Many people after knee replacement shorten terminal stance because stiffness, weakness, swelling, or reduced confidence make it feel uncomfortable to move fully over the foot. Instead of rolling forward smoothly, they may take a shorter step and move more cautiously.

That can produce:

- Shorter steps
- Reduced walking speed
- Reduced push-off power
- A stiff or shuffling walking pattern

Pre-Swing

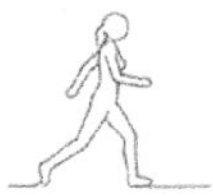

Pre-swing is the short transition period where the foot prepares to leave the ground. The body has already moved forward over the foot, and the leg is getting ready to swing through for the next step. The drawing illustrates this phase of walking, with the right leg closest to you serving as the reference leg.

During this phase:

- The toes remain briefly on the ground
- The knee begins bending
- The ankle helps create push-off into the next step

The calf muscles and ankle become major contributors during this phase. Ankle strength contributes far more to walking than most people realize because it helps create push-off, stride length, walking speed, and overall efficiency.

People recovering from knee replacement often avoid pushing fully through the foot because it feels stiff, unstable, or tiring. When push-off is reduced, walking may look shorter, flatter, or more cautious.

Weakness or hesitation during pre-swing can contribute to:

- Reduced push-off
- Shorter steps
- Shuffling
- Reduced walking rhythm

Swing Phase

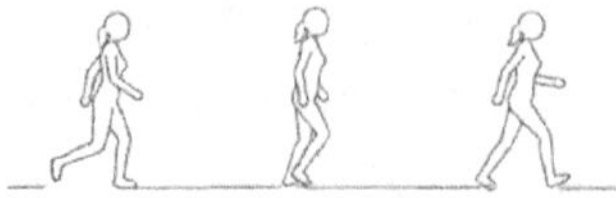

The swing phase is the part of walking when the foot leaves the ground, and the leg moves forward to prepare for the next step. This phase requires the hip to bring the leg forward, the knee to bend and then straighten, and the foot to clear the floor.

After knee replacement, swing phase may feel stiff or awkward when knee motion, hip strength, coordination, or confidence are limited. Some people compensate by hiking the hip, swinging the leg outward, shortening the step, or moving more cautiously than usual.

Initial Swing

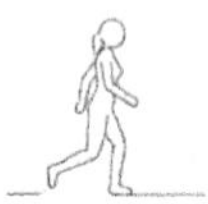

Initial swing begins once the foot leaves the ground and the leg starts moving forward. The goal is to clear the foot from the floor without dragging or catching the toes. The drawing illustrates this phase of walking, with the right leg closest to you serving as the reference leg.

During this phase:

- The knee bends to help lift the foot off the ground
- The hip begins moving the leg forward
- The foot clears the floor

Hip flexor strength, knee motion, and coordination all contribute during initial swing. If the knee remains too stiff, people may begin compensating by hiking the hip or swinging the leg outward instead of letting the leg move forward naturally.

Mid-Swing

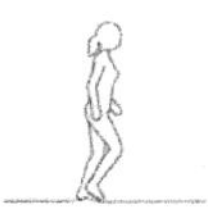

During mid-swing, the leg continues moving forward while the foot remains clear of the ground. The body is preparing the leg for the next step, and the knee gradually begins moving toward a straighter position. The drawing illustrates this phase of walking, with the right leg closest to you serving as the reference leg.

During this phase:

- The knee begins gradually straightening
- The hip continues advancing the leg forward
- The foot clears the floor as the body moves ahead

This phase helps position the leg for the next heel contact. If coordination, knee motion, or foot clearance are limited, people may shuffle, shorten the step, or drag the foot slightly.

Terminal Swing

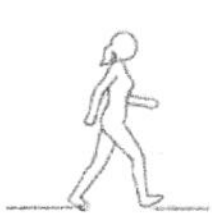

During terminal swing, the leg prepares for the next heel strike. This is the final part of swing phase before the foot contacts the ground again. The drawing illustrates this phase of walking, with the right leg closest to you serving as the reference leg.

During this phase:

- The knee straightens in preparation for weight acceptance
- The hip remains flexed forward
- The foot prepares for heel contact again

The muscles prepare the leg to accept weight again. If the knee does not straighten adequately before initial contact, people often begin landing more flat-footed or with a bent-knee walking pattern.

Common compensations include:

- Shortened stride length
- Stiff-leg movement
- Cautious foot placement
- Reduced walking rhythm

What Your Knee Is Doing During Walking

The knee acts as both a shock absorber and a stabilizer during walking. To move smoothly, it must repeatedly transition between mobility and stability within fractions of a second while the body moves from one leg to the other.

At initial contact, the leg approaches near full extension to prepare for efficient weight acceptance. As weight transfers onto the limb during loading response, the knee bends slightly to absorb force and reduce impact transmission. The quadriceps help control this motion while stabilizing the joint so the body can continue moving forward smoothly.

As the body progresses into mid-stance, the knee gradually straightens again. Physical therapists often refer to this as terminal knee extension, which means the knee reaches a position that is very close to fully straight while the body moves over the leg. This position is extremely important for efficient gait mechanics because it allows the body to move forward with less muscular effort and lower energy demand.

Loss of terminal knee extension after knee replacement often produces major gait changes. Even small extension deficits can contribute to:

- Persistent limping
- Reduced stride length
- Quadriceps inhibition

- Increased fatigue
- Compensatory hip and trunk movements
- Higher energy expenditure during walking

During swing phase, the knee flexes again to allow foot clearance. The knee then re-extends in preparation for the next step.

In many ways, normal gait depends on the knee repeatedly moving through a controlled cycle of:

- Extension for stability
- Flexion for shock absorption
- Extension for support
- Flexion for limb advancement

That cycle must occur smoothly and repeatedly for walking to feel natural.

Mobility And Joint Motion That Influence Walking

Walking requires more than strength alone. The hip, knee, and ankle also need enough motion to allow the body to move smoothly from one step to the next.

After knee replacement, stiffness and motion loss often change the way people walk long before strength fully returns. Even relatively small motion restrictions can create noticeable changes in stride length, push-off, walking rhythm, balance, and overall walking efficiency.

Certain movement limitations tend to influence walking more than others after knee replacement.

Knee Extension

Knee extension refers to the ability to fully straighten the knee.

This is one of the most important motions involved in walking.

During mid-stance, the knee normally moves very close to fully straight as the body passes over the leg. When full extension is limited, people often develop:

- Bent-knee walking
- Shorter stride length
- Increased fatigue
- Limping
- Reduced walking efficiency

Even small extension limitations can change walking mechanics significantly because the muscles must work harder during every step.

Knee Flexion

Knee flexion refers to bending the knee.

The knee bends during loading response to absorb force and again during swing phase to help the foot clear the floor.

When knee flexion feels stiff or restricted, walking may begin feeling:

- Robotic
- Stiff
- Less fluid
- More effortful

People may also compensate by hiking the hip, swinging the leg outward, or taking shorter steps.

Many people become highly focused on their range-of-motion numbers after surgery without fully understanding how those numbers relate to everyday walking.

For level-surface walking, the knee generally needs to reach close to full extension (around 0°) along with roughly 60° of knee flexion for a reasonably normal gait pattern.

Stairs and curbs usually require more motion.

Walking up and down stairs using a step-over-step pattern often requires roughly 90-120° of knee flexion depending on step height, speed, strength, balance, and individual walking mechanics. Curbs and uneven environments often require additional motion as well.

These ranges are broad functional estimates rather than strict requirements, and walking ability is influenced by many factors beyond range of motion alone. Individual mobility goals and walking progression should always be discussed with your surgeon or physical therapist.

This is one reason many people notice they can walk reasonably well on flat ground while still struggling with:

- Stairs
- Curbs
- Hills
- Low surfaces
- Getting in and out of cars

This does not necessarily mean progress has stopped. Different activities place different mobility demands on the knee.

Hip Extension

Hip extension occurs when the leg moves behind the body during walking.

This motion becomes especially important during terminal stance as the body moves forward over the foot.

Limited hip extension often contributes to:

- Shorter steps
- Reduced push-off
- Slower walking speed
- A more cautious walking pattern

Many people after knee replacement unconsciously shorten this phase because of stiffness, weakness, fatigue, or reduced confidence.

Ankle Motion

The ankle helps the body roll forward smoothly during walking and contributes significantly to push-off.

When ankle mobility becomes restricted, people often develop:

- Shorter steps
- Reduced push-off
- Flatter foot contact
- Slower walking speed
- A more shuffling walking pattern

Ankle stiffness and reduced push-off commonly become more noticeable during longer walks or when fatigue builds later in the day.

Muscle Groups That Influence Walking

After surgery, many people naturally focus almost entirely on the knee itself at first. But walking depends on much more than the knee alone.

Normal gait requires strength, coordination, balance, and timing throughout the entire lower body. Different muscle groups contribute to balance, weight acceptance, stability, forward movement, and walking efficiency during different parts of each step.

When one muscle group becomes weak, stiff, fatigued, or poorly coordinated, the entire walking pattern often changes. Understanding which muscles contribute to walking can help people better understand why certain walking changes develop and why different exercises target different problems.

Some muscle groups tend to influence walking more noticeably after knee replacement than others. The sections below move from larger walking muscles and common gait contributors toward smaller support muscles involved in balance and foot control.

Quadriceps

The quadriceps are the large muscles on the front of the thigh.

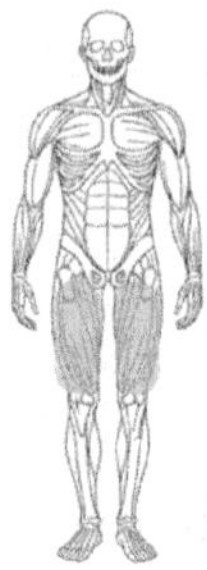

They help:

- Control knee bending
- Stabilize the leg during weight acceptance
- Support mid-stance stability
- Assist with stair climbing

Weak quadriceps often contribute to limping and reduced confidence.

Gluteus Medius

The gluteus medius is a hip muscle located along the outer side of the pelvis.

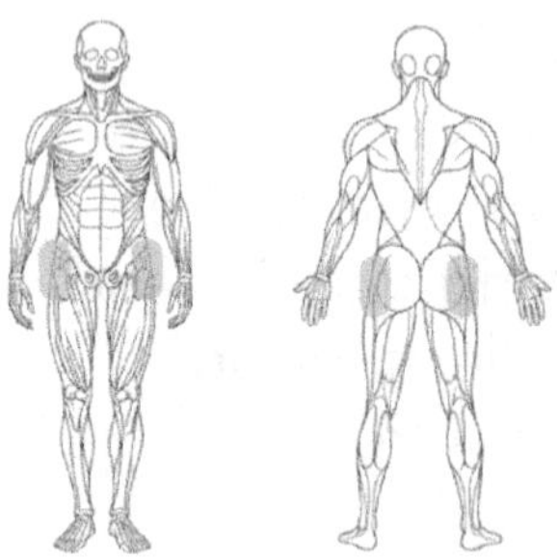

This muscle stabilizes the pelvis during single-leg standing.

Weakness here often contributes to:

- Trunk leaning
- Hip drop
- Side-to-side walking
- Balance problems

Gluteus Maximus

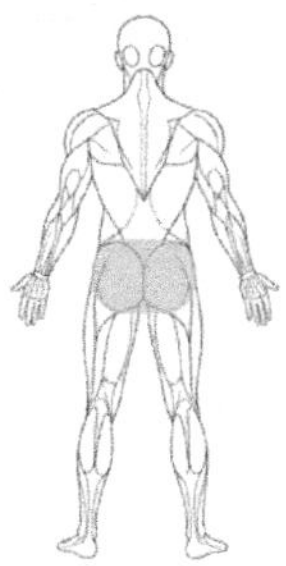

The gluteus maximus is the large muscle at the back of the hip and buttock region.

This muscle helps control hip extension and upright posture during walking.

Tightness, weakness, or poor coordination here can contribute to:

- Forward lean of trunk
- Flexed posture

Hamstrings

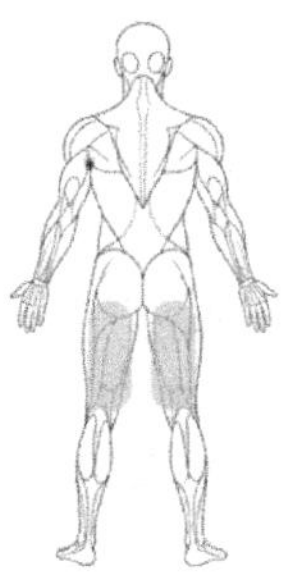

The hamstrings are located along the back of the thigh.

These muscles help bend the knee and assist with controlling the leg during walking.

Tightness, weakness, or poor coordination here can contribute to:

- Difficulty fully straightening the knee
- Shortened stride length
- Stiffness during walking
- Reduced walking rhythm

Hip Flexors

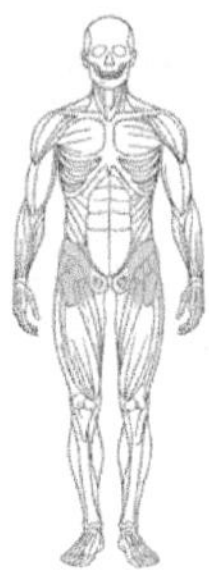

The hip flexors are located along the front of the hip and upper thigh.

These muscles help lift the leg and move it forward during walking.

Weakness or fatigue here can contribute to:

- Shorter steps
- Slower walking speed
- Difficulty lifting the leg during swing phase
- Increased effort during stairs or curbs

Trunk and Core Muscles

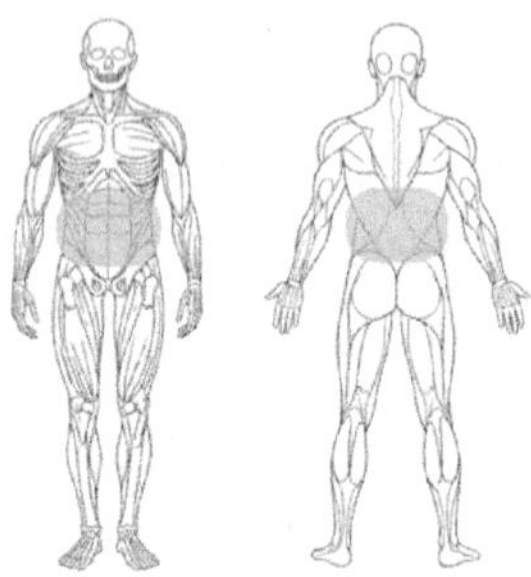

The trunk and core muscles include the abdominal muscles, back extensors, and deeper stabilizing muscles around the pelvis and spine.

These muscles help maintain upright posture, balance, and stability while walking.

When trunk control becomes fatigued or less coordinated, people often begin leaning more, walking more cautiously, or losing smooth walking rhythm.

Calf Muscles

The calf muscles are located on the back of the lower leg.

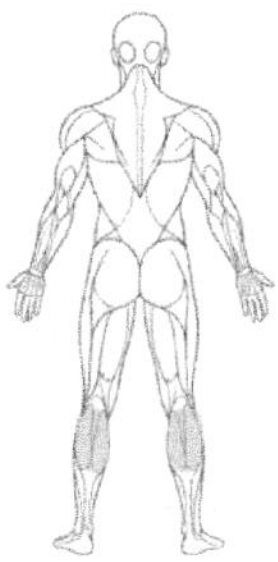

The calf muscles create push-off power.

Weakness here often reduces walking speed and efficiency.

Ankle Muscles

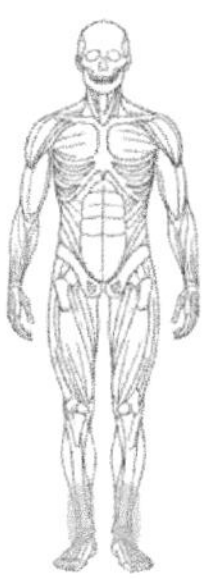

The ankle muscles surround the lower leg and ankle region.

The ankle muscles help control foot placement, balance, stability, and coordination throughout walking.

Weakness, stiffness, or poor coordination here can contribute to:

- Balance problems
- Poor foot placement
- Shuffling
- Difficulty walking on uneven surfaces
- Reduced walking confidence
- Slower walking speed

REBUILDING STRENGTH FOR WALKING

Improving walking after knee replacement usually requires more than simply forcing yourself to walk farther. Walking quality often improves more steadily when strength, endurance, balance, coordination, and confidence all improve together over time.

Different exercises target different muscle groups involved in walking. Most rehabilitation programs combine several types of exercises together because walking depends on many body systems working together smoothly.

Strengthening exercises are usually most helpful when gains in strength gradually carry over into real-world walking activities such as navigating stairs, changing direction, walking outdoors, and moving through everyday environments.

The examples below are commonly used in rehabilitation programs, but not every exercise is appropriate for every individual or every stage after surgery.

Exercise selection and progression should be individualized based on mobility, strength, balance, pain levels, surgical history, and guidance from your healthcare team.

Quadriceps

Common exercises used to strengthen the quadriceps include:

- Sit-to-stands
- Step-ups
- Knee extension exercises

These exercises help improve weight acceptance, stair climbing, and knee stability during walking.

Gluteus Medius

Common exercises used to strengthen the gluteus medius include:

- Side-stepping exercises
- Standing hip abduction
- Single-leg balance exercises

These exercises help improve pelvic stability, balance, and control during single-leg standing.

Gluteus Maximus

Common exercises used to strengthen the gluteus maximus include:

- Bridges
- Sit-to-stands
- Stair climbing exercises

These exercises help improve upright posture, forward movement, and walking power.

Hamstrings

Common exercises used to strengthen the hamstrings include:

- Romanian deadlifts
- Standing hamstring curls
- Step-up variations

These exercises help support knee control and improve walking rhythm.

Hip Flexors

Common exercises used to strengthen the hip flexors include:

- Marching exercises
- Step-over drills
- Resisted hip flexion exercises

These exercises help improve leg advancement and foot clearance during walking.

Trunk and Core Muscles

Common exercises used to improve trunk and core control include:

- Planks
- Squatting exercises
- Bridging exercises

These exercises help improve posture, balance, walking stability, and overall movement control.

Calf Muscles

Common exercises used to strengthen the calf muscles include:

- Heel raises
- Stair climbing exercises
- Walking uphill

These exercises help improve push-off strength and walking efficiency.

Ankle Muscles

Common exercises used to improve ankle strength and control include:

- Balance exercises
- Heel-toe walking
- Resisted ankle exercises

These exercises help improve foot placement, walking stability, and balance on uneven surfaces.

The goal is usually not perfect exercise performance. More often, progress develops through repeated practice, manageable effort, and gradual improvement over time.

Many people also benefit from working with a physical therapist to identify which muscle groups need the most attention and to build a more targeted walking and strengthening program.

How Walking Patterns Adapt After Knee Replacement

Earlier in this guide, we talked about how limping and walking changes are often influenced by swelling, fatigue, weakness, confidence, and protective movement patterns rather than one isolated problem. Walking changes are usually influenced by several factors interacting together at the same time.

As these factors build on each other, walking rhythm often becomes less automatic and more compensatory. Some of the most common patterns involve swelling, fatigue, stiffness, weakness, and cautious movement gradually accumulating throughout the day. A person may start the morning walking fairly comfortably, then notice increasing stiffness and fatigue after longer activity. As the leg tires, coordination and confidence often decrease further, which can make limping or compensations more noticeable later in the day. Overdoing activity early can sometimes create a snowball effect where swelling, fatigue, stiffness, and walking changes all become more noticeable together afterward.

Common contributors include:

- Swelling
- Weakness
- Reduced knee extension
- Fatigue
- Altered balance
- Confidence changes

- Compensation patterns
- Loss of walking rhythm

Small adjustments earlier in the day can often prevent several of these factors from building on each other later. Pacing activity more evenly, taking short movement breaks, managing swelling early, and avoiding the urge to overdo "good days" can sometimes reduce the buildup of fatigue, stiffness, swelling, and compensation patterns before they begin stacking together.

Carol eventually realized that smooth walking was not about forcing herself to walk perfectly. It was about rebuilding the pieces that allow walking to become automatic again.

Once she became more proactive about pacing activity, managing swelling, rebuilding strength, and paying attention to fatigue earlier, walking started feeling more natural and less exhausting throughout the day.

As strength improved, swelling decreased, and confidence returned, her gait became smoother without obsessing over every single step.

That is often how walking improves after knee replacement.

Not through perfect walking immediately, but through gradual restoration of rhythm, coordination, confidence, endurance, and movement quality.

Walking Support And Movement Quality

Using a walker or cane after knee replacement can bring up strong feelings for many people. Support devices are often emotionally connected to aging, weakness, dependence, or loss of independence, even though many people continue living active and fully independent lives while using them.

The goal is not simply walking without support. The goal is walking more smoothly, safely, and efficiently with the right amount of support when needed. In many cases, the right support device allows people to stay more active, walk longer distances more comfortably, participate in more activities, and move through the community with greater confidence, better balance, and less fatigue. Without enough support, people often begin compensating more heavily, avoiding activities, or tiring much faster.

Rather than limiting independence, the right amount of support often helps people stay engaged in daily life while strength, endurance, balance, and walking quality continue improving.

Carol struggled with this for a while. She disliked bringing the cane into public places and worried people would view her differently. At home she sometimes tried walking without it simply to prove to herself that she could.

What eventually changed her perspective was realizing that she actually walked better with the cane than without it.

With the cane:

- Her stride became smoother
- Her limp decreased
- Her posture improved
- Her balance improved
- Her walking rhythm improved
- She felt more relaxed
- Longer walks became less tiring

Without it, she often compensated heavily and became fatigued much faster.

That realization helped her stop viewing the cane as a sign of failure and start viewing it as temporary support that allowed her to move more smoothly and with less fatigue.

As walking quality improves, the transition away from the cane often happens naturally. Signs people often look for include:

- Less limping throughout the day
- Improved balance
- More consistent endurance
- Smoother weight shifting
- Less fatigue during longer walks
- Greater confidence in public settings

One question eventually helped Carol think about the cane differently:

"Do I walk better with the cane than without it?"

If the answer is yes, the cane may still be helping your body move more naturally while strength, confidence, and endurance continue improving.

Common Walking Habits That Can Slow Progress

There are several patterns that consistently create frustration while people are learning to walk more naturally again.

One of the most common is turning good days into marathon activity days. Carol would start feeling better and suddenly decide to clean the house, grocery shop, reorganize cabinets, and stay on her feet for hours. Later that evening or the next day, walking often became more difficult again because her knee was more painful, swollen, and stiff.

Another common pattern is continuing to walk long after walking becomes more uneven and compensation patterns begin increasing. Many people keep pushing through obvious fatigue because they assume more walking automatically means faster progress. In reality, walking quality often matters more than total distance.

People also frequently abandon their cane too early. In many cases, the decision has less to do with walking quality and more to do with what the cane feels like it represents emotionally. Some people dislike the attention it brings in public or worry it means they are not progressing fast enough, even when the cane is still improving rhythm, confidence, balance, and overall walking quality.

At the same time, some people continue relying heavily on the cane long after walking quality and balance have improved enough to begin practicing more unsupported walking in safe environments. In some cases, this can unintentionally reinforce uneven weight shifting or cautious walking patterns. The goal is usually not getting rid of support as fast as possible or holding onto it unnecessarily long. The goal is using the amount of support that helps walking feel smooth, stable, and efficient while confidence and strength continue improving.

Over-monitoring movement can also become a habit that makes walking feel more difficult. Some people focus so intensely on every step that walking becomes stiff and unnatural. Others become discouraged by comparing their progress to someone else online or in physical therapy.

Walking after surgery rarely improves in a perfectly straight line. Most people experience a mix of stronger days, stiff days, fatigue days, swelling days, and frustrating days along the way. Constantly analyzing every difficult walk or temporary setback often increases tension, frustration, and self-conscious movement patterns instead of allowing walking to become more relaxed and natural.

Over time, many people begin recognizing that these habits are often driven by frustration, impatience, fear, comparison, or the desire to get back to normal as quickly as possible. The encouraging part is that walking habits can change. Small adjustments in pacing, support use, activity balance, and expectations often help walking feel smoother, more natural, and less mentally draining.

When Walking Stops Feeling Automatic

Walking after knee replacement is not purely mechanical. Confidence, attention, environment, and self-consciousness can all change the way people move.

Many people notice they walk differently in crowded stores, unfamiliar environments, around strangers, or anytime they feel rushed or uncertain. Walking that feels fairly natural at home may suddenly become more cautious and stiff in busy public environments.

Carol gradually realized she walked very differently in public than she did at home. Part of it was physical, but part of it was also the uncomfortable feeling of not moving as naturally or keeping pace with other people the way she used to.

I once spoke with a woman whose daughter kept mentioning that she was limping. At first she did not think her walking looked very different. Later, she happened to watch footage from her doorbell camera and immediately noticed how stiff and cautious she looked while walking.

Seeing herself on video helped her understand why walking had started feeling so tiring and unnatural during public outings.

At home she relaxed more and moved more automatically without thinking about every step. Outside she became more self-conscious, especially when trying to keep pace with other people or move through crowded public spaces.

This is extremely common after surgery. The nervous system often becomes more protective when people feel fatigued, rushed, uncertain, or less confident in unfamiliar environments. As tension increases, walking frequently becomes stiffer, shorter, slower, and less automatic.

Confidence usually rebuilds gradually through repetition, familiarity, successful experiences, improving endurance, and repeated exposure to normal daily activities. Most people do not suddenly wake up feeling fully confident again. More often, walking slowly begins feeling less mentally demanding and more natural again.

Over time, the nervous system gradually relearns smoother, more efficient movement patterns.

Relearning Smoother Walking Patterns

Walking patterns often improve through repetition and motor learning. As strength, endurance, balance, and mobility improve, walking often starts feeling smoother, more coordinated, and more confident over time. In some cases, the body continues repeating protective walking patterns even after swelling, weakness, or discomfort begin improving because those movement habits have become more automatic over time.

For some people, skilled gait assessment and walking retraining from a physical therapist can be extremely valuable, especially when limping, asymmetrical walking patterns, balance problems, or compensations remain noticeable later after surgery.

Building Walking Tolerance Over Time

One of the hardest parts of rebuilding walking tolerance is realizing that the body often handles short periods of walking much better than long periods of continuous activity.

Many people begin feeling more comfortable indoors and assume they are ready for long outings, grocery stores, vacations, crowded environments, or extended time on their feet. Then later that day or the following morning, they suddenly notice increased swelling, stiffness, limping, or fatigue.

Outdoor and community walking often involve much longer continuous movement, uneven surfaces, stairs, curbs, standing without breaks, distractions, turns, and constantly changing environments. These situations often become tiring faster than people expect, especially during the earlier stages after surgery.

Carol experienced this repeatedly during the first several months after surgery. On days she felt stronger, she often tried to make up for lost time. She would run errands, stay active for hours, and push herself because she wanted life to feel normal again.

The problem was not usually one specific activity. More often, the entire day added up.

Eventually she noticed something important. When activity stayed reasonably consistent from day to day, walking began improving more steadily. Swelling became easier to manage, fatigue became less dramatic, and walking started feeling smoother and less effortful.

Many people notice similar improvements when they:

- Build walking time steadily instead of making huge jumps
- Start with shorter outings before attempting longer ones
- Rest before severe fatigue develops

- Reduce activity temporarily when swelling, limping, or fatigue begin building up
- Keep activity reasonably consistent from day to day

As strength and endurance improve, people often gradually begin returning to activities they care deeply about.

Sometimes that means walking through the grocery store comfortably again. For others it means traveling, attending social events, walking through parks with family members, or returning to hiking trails they had stopped enjoying before surgery.

Carol eventually returned to a local walking trail she used to avoid because of pain and instability before surgery. She still noticed some stiffness afterward and occasionally needed to slow down or take short breaks along the trail.

But something about the experience felt different.

Walking did not need to feel perfect for life to start feeling bigger again.

She was moving through life again instead of organizing life around her knee.

When To Contact Your Healthcare Team

Most walking changes after knee replacement are expected and improve gradually over time. At the same time, certain symptoms or sudden changes should not be ignored.

The examples below are not a complete list, but they are situations where contacting your surgeon or healthcare team may be important.

Examples include:

- Sudden inability to bear weight
- Major increase in swelling
- Increasing redness or drainage
- Severe calf pain
- Sudden major decline in walking ability
- New neurological symptoms
- Chest pain or shortness of breath
- Major pain after a fall

If something feels significantly different from your usual pattern or symptoms are worsening unexpectedly, contact your healthcare provider.

Quick Reference: Common Walking Changes After Knee Replacement

Walking Change	What It May Feel Like	Common Contributing Factors	What Often Helps
Slower walking speed	Walking feels slower than expected, or it becomes hard to keep pace with others	reduced quadriceps and hip strength, shorter step length, reduced push-off, pain, swelling, balance concerns, reduced confidence	strengthening, gradual walking practice, balance work, pacing, support when it improves walking quality
Reduced walking endurance	Short walks feel manageable, but longer outings become tiring quickly	reduced conditioning, muscle fatigue, swelling buildup, pain, balance demands, too much activity at once	shorter activity bursts, planned breaks, gradual endurance building, consistent activity levels,

Walking Change	What It May Feel Like	Common Contributing Factors	What Often Helps
			pacing before fatigue builds
Bent-knee walking	The knee does not feel fully straight during standing or walking	loss of terminal knee extension, swelling, quadriceps weakness, pain, protective movement patterns	knee extension mobility, quadriceps strengthening, gait practice, swelling management, confident weight bearing
Reduced knee bending during walking	The knee feels stiff, robotic, or less responsive during each step	swelling, stiffness, pain, quadriceps inhibition, stiffness with bending the knee during walking	swelling management, mobility work, strengthening, gait practice with a physical therapist
Shorter step or stride length	Steps feel smaller, slower,	limited knee extension, pain, stiffness, reduced push-	improving knee extension and push-off,

Walking Change	What It May Feel Like	Common Contributing Factors	What Often Helps
	cautious, or uneven	off, cautious walking patterns, reduced confidence	gradual walking practice, rhythm and stride practice, pacing, support when helpful
Reduced push-off	Walking feels slower, heavier, shuffling, or less fluid	calf weakness, ankle stiffness, shortened terminal stance, cautious weight transfer, reduced confidence	calf strengthening, ankle mobility, gradual walking practice, improving forward weight transfer during walking
Longer double-support time or cautious weight shifting	More time spent with both feet on the ground or hesitation	balance changes, pain, quadriceps weakness, reduced trust	balance work, gradual weight-shifting practice, confident

Walking Change	What It May Feel Like	Common Contributing Factors	What Often Helps
	loading the surgical leg	in the leg, fear of instability	single-leg loading, support device if it improves walking quality
Side-to-side shifting or trunk lean	More leaning, side-to-side motion, or uneven weight shifting while walking	hip weakness, balance changes, reduced trust in the leg, reduced stance time on the surgical leg	hip strengthening, balance work, cane use if it improves walking quality
Flat-foot contact or reduced heel strike	Foot lands flatter instead of rolling smoothly from heel to toe	limited knee extension, short cautious steps, ankle stiffness, difficulty fully straightening the knee before stepping	gait practice, ankle mobility, knee extension work, heel-first walking practice when appropriate

Walking Change	What It May Feel Like	Common Contributing Factors	What Often Helps
Reduced cadence (slower step rhythm)	Steps feel slower and less continuous	fatigue, stiffness, shorter stride length, cautious movement, balance concerns	gradual walking practice with steady rhythm, strengthening, pacing
Stiff first steps	First steps after sitting feel tight or awkward	swelling, stiffness, limited motion, stiffness after sitting or inactivity	avoid sitting too long at one time, swelling management, gentle warm-up
Fatigue-related limping	Walking starts comfortably, then limping gradually increases later in the day	muscle fatigue, endurance limits, swelling buildup, overdoing activity	pacing, shorter outings, planned rest breaks, gradual endurance building
Difficulty adapting to	Walking feels less steady	balance changes,	balance training, stair

Walking Change	What It May Feel Like	Common Contributing Factors	What Often Helps
uneven or changing environments	on curbs, stairs, uneven ground, turns, or busy environments	reduced confidence, slower balance reactions, weakness, reduced automatic movement	practice, uneven surface walking, walking practice in changing environments, gradually spending more time in community environments
Walking feels mentally demanding	Walking requires constant attention, especially in public or busy environments	self-consciousness, walking no longer feels automatic, protective tension, balance concerns, fatigue	repetition, confidence building, walking in progressively busier environments, walking while gradually doing more than one thing at a time

Walking Change	What It May Feel Like	Common Contributing Factors	What Often Helps
Walking feels stiffer in public	Walking feels worse in stores or busy environments	self-consciousness, tension, confidence changes, feeling rushed or observed, uneven surfaces	repetition, familiar environments, pacing, support when helpful
Overdoing good days	Knee feels worse later that day or the next day	too much activity, swelling buildup, fatigue building up, long periods on feet	consistent activity levels, shorter activity bursts, planned breaks

This quick reference chart is not all-inclusive. Walking changes after knee replacement vary significantly between individuals depending on strength, swelling, balance, mobility, pain levels, overall conditioning, surgical history, and other medical factors.

Try not to focus on fixing everything at once. Most people do better when they identify one or two walking issues that seem most noticeable and gradually work on those areas over time.

If you are unsure what your walking pattern actually looks like, it can sometimes help to have someone record a short video of you walking from the front, side, and behind. Watching a short video often helps people notice walking patterns more objectively.

Walking quality often changes from one day to the next. In many cases, progress develops gradually through repetition, consistency, pacing, and giving yourself time to adapt rather than expecting every walk to feel perfect.

Movement Does Not Need To Be Perfect

The human body is remarkably adaptable. Many people continue noticing small asymmetries, stiffness, or movement differences long after surgery, yet still return to traveling, shopping, social activities, exercise, and everyday life. No one walks perfectly all day long. Even healthy walking naturally changes depending on fatigue, stress, speed, terrain, distractions, soreness, footwear, energy level, and countless other factors.

After knee replacement, many people become highly aware of every step. They start monitoring whether they are limping, thinking about how their walking looks in public, or worrying that every awkward movement means something is wrong. In many cases, the harder people try to consciously control every step, the less automatic walking begins to feel.

That does not mean walking mechanics are unimportant. Strength, balance, mobility, endurance, and walking quality still play important roles. But many people eventually improve more by gradually rebuilding trust, repetition, confidence, and participation in daily life than by obsessing over whether every single step looks perfect.

Many people eventually stop focusing so heavily on whether every step looks exactly right. Over time, walking often starts feeling more natural again as people rebuild trust in their body, spend more time participating in normal life, and stop treating every awkward step like a sign that something is wrong.

Final Thoughts

Walking after knee replacement is often influenced by far more than the knee itself. Swelling, fatigue, strength, confidence, and activity levels are constantly changing, which is one reason walking can feel very different from one day to the next.

Walking improvements are usually not built through one perfect week of rehabilitation or one major breakthrough moment. More often, they develop through repetition, pacing, rebuilding confidence, and hundreds of ordinary walks repeated over time.

Understanding your walking patterns is very different than obsessing over every step. In many cases, people improve more steadily once they can recognize fatigue, swelling, and activity buildup without treating every difficult walking day like something has gone wrong.

And over time, many people eventually notice a shift.

They spend less time thinking about their knee and more time simply participating in life again.

Continue Learning With Total Knee Success

If this guide helped you better understand what you may be experiencing after knee replacement surgery, you can find additional educational resources at:

TotalKneeSuccess.com

There you'll find:

- The Total Knee Success Podcast™
- Other books: Making Sense of Pain After Knee Replacement.
- The Total Knee Success™ Insider Newsletter sign-up, where you get ongoing educational content designed to support people at different stages after surgery.

Scan to visit totalkneesuccess.com

If this guide was helpful to you, leaving a review on Amazon helps other knee replacement patients find the information they may be looking for.

Thank you for supporting Total Knee Success™.

About The Author

Michelle Losurdo, PT, DPT, Board-certified Orthopedic Clinical Specialist, is a physical therapist specializing in total knee replacement rehabilitation.

She is the creator and host of the Total Knee Success Podcast, where she helps knee replacement patients better understand pain, stiffness, swelling, walking, sleep, and the realities of rehabilitation after surgery.

Known for her calm, practical, evidence-informed approach, Michelle translates complex rehabilitation concepts into language people can actually use in daily life.

Her goal is simple: helping people better understand what they're experiencing so they can move forward with more clarity, confidence, and success after knee replacement.

Visit TotalKneeSuccess.com for additional resources, podcast episodes, and educational guides.

REFERENCES

The following sources reflect key research and clinical concepts that inform the ideas presented in this guide. They are provided for those who want to explore the topics in more depth.

Alnahdi AH, Zeni JA Jr, Snyder-Mackler L. Gait after unilateral total knee arthroplasty: frontal plane analysis. Phys Ther. 2011;91(5):647-657. doi:10.2522/ptj.20100323

Bade MJ, Stevens-Lapsley JE. Restoration of physical function in patients following total knee arthroplasty: an update on rehabilitation practices. Clin Geriatr Med. 2012;28(3):489-500. doi:10.1016/j.cger.2012.05.001

Benedetti MG, Catani F, Bilotta TW, et al. Muscle activation pattern and gait biomechanics after total knee replacement. Clin Biomech (Bristol, Avon). 2003;18(9):871-876. doi:10.1016/S0268-0033(03)00146-3

Boukabache A, Maruthainar N, Manhas V, Player D. Multidimensional Assessment of Recovery After Total Knee Arthroplasty in Clinical Practice: Critical Narrative Review. JMIR Perioper Med. 2026;9:e84011. doi:10.2196/84011

Capin JJ, Bade MJ, Jennings JM, Snyder-Mackler L, Stevens-Lapsley JE. Total knee arthroplasty assessments should include strength and performance-based functional tests to complement range-of-motion and patient-reported outcome measures. Phys Ther. 2022;102(6):pzac033. doi:10.1093/ptj/pzac033

Capin JJ, Zeni JA Jr, Forster JE, et al. Preoperative and Post-Rehabilitation Predictors of Gait Biomechanics Six Months After Total Knee Arthroplasty. J Orthop Res. 2025;43(11):1964-1972. doi:10.1002/jor.70052

Christiansen CL, Bade MJ, Davidson BS, Dayton MR, Stevens-Lapsley JE. Effects of weight-bearing biofeedback training on functional movement patterns following total knee arthroplasty: a randomized controlled trial. J Orthop Sports Phys Ther. 2015;45(9):647-655. doi:10.2519/jospt.2015.5595

Farquhar SJ, Snyder-Mackler L. The Chitranjan Ranawat Award: the nonoperated knee predicts function 3 years after unilateral total knee arthroplasty. Clin Orthop Relat Res. 2010;468(1):37-44. doi:10.1007/s11999-009-0911-y

Heckmann TP, Fleckenstein C, Noyes FR. Total Knee Arthroplasty Rehabilitation Strategies for Avoiding Arthrofibrosis and Other Complications with the Goal of Return to Recreational Activities and Active Lifestyle. Int J Sports Phys Ther. 2026;21(2):173-183. doi:10.26603/001c.155480

Jette DU, Hunter SJ, Burkett L, et al. Physical therapist management of total knee arthroplasty. Phys Ther. 2020;100(9):1603-1631. doi:10.1093/ptj/pzaa099

Karimijashni M, Yoo S, Barnes K, et al. Postoperative Rehabilitation Interventions in Patients at Risk of Poorer Outcomes Following Total Knee Arthroplasty: A

Systematic Review. Musculoskeletal Care. 2025;23(1):e70054. doi:10.1002/msc.70054

Konnyu KJ, Thoma LM, Cao W, et al. Rehabilitation for Total Knee Arthroplasty: A Systematic Review. Am J Phys Med Rehabil. 2023;102(1):19-33. doi:10.1097/PHM.0000000000002008

Mandeville D, Osternig LR, Chou LS. The effect of total knee replacement on dynamic support of the body during walking and stair ascent. Clin Biomech (Bristol, Avon). 2008;23(6):787-794. doi:10.1016/j.clinbiomech.2008.02.011

Marino G, De Capitani F, Adamo P, Bolzoni L, Gatti R, Temporiti F. Long-term gait analysis in patients after total knee arthroplasty: A systematic review and meta-analysis. Gait Posture. 2024;113:75-98. doi:10.1016/j.gaitpost.2024.06.002

McClelland JA, Webster KE, Feller JA. Gait analysis of patients following total knee replacement: a systematic review. Knee. 2007;14(4):253-263. doi:10.1016/j.knee.2007.04.008

Mizner RL, Petterson SC, Snyder-Mackler L. Quadriceps strength and the time course of functional recovery after total knee arthroplasty. J Orthop Res. 2005;23(2):424-430. doi:10.1016/j.orthres.2004.07.004

Nanjo K, Ikeda T, Kaneyama R, Okuyama H, Sakai T, Jinno T. Criteria for knee flexion range of motion and quadriceps strength to ascend and descend stairs 1 year after bilateral total knee arthroplasty: A cross-sectional study. J Back Musculoskelet Rehabil. 2025;38(5). doi:10.1177/10538127251323980

National Institute for Health and Care Excellence. Joint replacement (primary): hip, knee and shoulder. NICE guideline NG157. Published June 2020. Accessed May 17, 2026. https://www.nice.org.uk/guidance/ng157

Pozzi F, Snyder-Mackler L, Zeni J Jr. Physical exercise after knee arthroplasty: a systematic review of controlled trials. Eur J Phys Rehabil Med. 2013;49(6):877-892.

Rosenberg N. Walking Ability After Total Knee Arthroplasty: A Comprehensive Review. Cureus. 2025;17(2):e79577. doi:10.7759/cureus.79577

Perry J, Burnfield JM. Gait Analysis: Normal and Pathological Function. 2nd ed. SLACK Incorporated; 2010.

Rancho Los Amigos National Rehabilitation Center. *Observational Gait Analysis.* 4th ed. Downey, CA: Los Amigos Research and Education Institute, Rancho Los Amigos National Rehabilitation Center; 2001.

Rowe PJ, Myles CM, Walker C, Nutton R. Knee joint kinematics in gait and other functional activities measured using flexible electrogoniometry: how much knee motion is necessary for normal daily life? Gait Posture. 2000;12(2):143-155. doi:10.1016/S0966-6362(00)00060-6

Walsh M, Woodhouse LJ, Thomas SG, Finch E. Physical impairments and functional limitations: a comparison of individuals 1 year after total knee arthroplasty with control subjects. Phys Ther. 1998;78(3):248-258. doi:10.1093/ptj/78.3.248

Wylde V, Beswick AD, Dennis J, Gooberman-Hill R. Chronic pain after total knee arthroplasty. EFORT Open Rev. 2018;3(8):461-470. doi:10.1302/2058-5241.3.180004

Zeni JA Jr, Snyder-Mackler L. Early postoperative measures predict 1- and 2-year outcomes after unilateral total knee arthroplasty. J Orthop Res. 2010;28(8):1021-1026. doi:10.1002/jor.21095

These references are included to support the general concepts discussed and are not required reading to benefit from this guide.

Made in the USA
Monee, IL
13 September 2026

62979550R00046